THIS BOOK BELONGS TO :

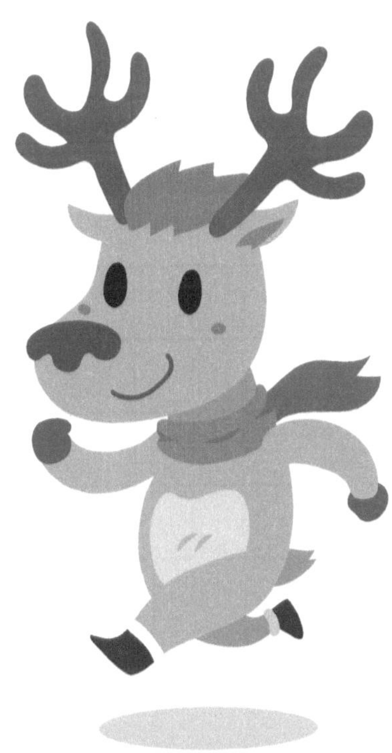

WEEK ....

DATE ....

Time	Monday	Tuesday	Wednesday	Thursday
Breakfast				
2 hr after				
Lunch				
2 hr after				
Dinner				
2 hr after				
Bedtime				

Time	Friday	Saturday	Sunday	NOTE
Breakfast				
2 hr after				
Lunch				
2 hr after				
Dinner				
2 hr after				
Bedtime				

WEEK ....

DATE ....

Time	Monday	Tuesday	Wednesday	Thursday
Breakfast				
2 hr after				
Lunch				
2 hr after				
Dinner				
2 hr after				
Bedtime				

Time	Friday	Saturday	Sunday	NOTE
Breakfast				
2 hr after				
Lunch				
2 hr after				
Dinner				
2 hr after				
Bedtime				

WEEK ....

DATE ....

Time	Monday	Tuesday	Wednesday	Thursday
Breakfast				
2 hr after				
Lunch				
2 hr after				
Dinner				
2 hr after				
Bedtime				

Time	Friday	Saturday	Sunday	NOTE
Breakfast				
2 hr after				
Lunch				
2 hr after				
Dinner				
2 hr after				
Bedtime				

WEEK ....

DATE ....

Time	Monday	Tuesday	Wednesday	Thursday
Breakfast				
2 hr after				
Lunch				
2 hr after				
Dinner				
2 hr after				
Bedtime				

Time	Friday	Saturday	Sunday	NOTE
Breakfast				
2 hr after				
Lunch				
2 hr after				
Dinner				
2 hr after				
Bedtime				

WEEK ....

DATE ....

Time	Monday	Tuesday	Wednesday	Thursday
Breakfast				
2 hr after				
Lunch				
2 hr after				
Dinner				
2 hr after				
Bedtime				

Time	Friday	Saturday	Sunday	NOTE
Breakfast				
2 hr after				
Lunch				
2 hr after				
Dinner				
2 hr after				
Bedtime				

WEEK ....

DATE ....

Time	Monday	Tuesday	Wednesday	Thursday
Breakfast				
2 hr after				
Lunch				
2 hr after				
Dinner				
2 hr after				
Bedtime				

Time	Friday	Saturday	Sunday	NOTE
Breakfast				
2 hr after				
Lunch				
2 hr after				
Dinner				
2 hr after				
Bedtime				

WEEK ....

DATE ....

Time	Monday	Tuesday	Wednesday	Thursday
Breakfast				
2 hr after				
Lunch				
2 hr after				
Dinner				
2 hr after				
Bedtime				

Time	Friday	Saturday	Sunday	NOTE
Breakfast				
2 hr after				
Lunch				
2 hr after				
Dinner				
2 hr after				
Bedtime				

WEEK ....

DATE ....

Time	Monday	Tuesday	Wednesday	Thursday
Breakfast				
2 hr after				
Lunch				
2 hr after				
Dinner				
2 hr after				
Bedtime				

Time	Friday	Saturday	Sunday	NOTE
Breakfast				
2 hr after				
Lunch				
2 hr after				
Dinner				
2 hr after				
Bedtime				

WEEK ....

DATE ....

Time	Monday	Tuesday	Wednesday	Thursday
Breakfast				
2 hr after				
Lunch				
2 hr after				
Dinner				
2 hr after				
Bedtime				

Time	Friday	Saturday	Sunday	NOTE
Breakfast				
2 hr after				
Lunch				
2 hr after				
Dinner				
2 hr after				
Bedtime				

WEEK ....

DATE ....

Time	Monday	Tuesday	Wednesday	Thursday
Breakfast				
2 hr after				
Lunch				
2 hr after				
Dinner				
2 hr after				
Bedtime				

Time	Friday	Saturday	Sunday	NOTE
Breakfast				
2 hr after				
Lunch				
2 hr after				
Dinner				
2 hr after				
Bedtime				

WEEK ....

DATE ....

Time	Monday	Tuesday	Wednesday	Thursday
Breakfast				
2 hr after				
Lunch				
2 hr after				
Dinner				
2 hr after				
Bedtime				

Time	Friday	Saturday	Sunday	NOTE
Breakfast				
2 hr after				
Lunch				
2 hr after				
Dinner				
2 hr after				
Bedtime				

WEEK ....

DATE ....

Time	Monday	Tuesday	Wednesday	Thursday
Breakfast				
2 hr after				
Lunch				
2 hr after				
Dinner				
2 hr after				
Bedtime				

Time	Friday	Saturday	Sunday	NOTE
Breakfast				
2 hr after				
Lunch				
2 hr after				
Dinner				
2 hr after				
Bedtime				

WEEK ....

DATE ....

Time	Monday	Tuesday	Wednesday	Thursday
Breakfast				
2 hr after				
Lunch				
2 hr after				
Dinner				
2 hr after				
Bedtime				

Time	Friday	Saturday	Sunday	NOTE
Breakfast				
2 hr after				
Lunch				
2 hr after				
Dinner				
2 hr after				
Bedtime				

WEEK ....

DATE ....

Time	Monday	Tuesday	Wednesday	Thursday
Breakfast				
2 hr after				
Lunch				
2 hr after				
Dinner				
2 hr after				
Bedtime				

Time	Friday	Saturday	Sunday	NOTE
Breakfast				
2 hr after				
Lunch				
2 hr after				
Dinner				
2 hr after				
Bedtime				

WEEK ....

DATE ....

Time	Monday	Tuesday	Wednesday	Thursday
Breakfast				
2 hr after				
Lunch				
2 hr after				
Dinner				
2 hr after				
Bedtime				

Time	Friday	Saturday	Sunday	NOTE
Breakfast				
2 hr after				
Lunch				
2 hr after				
Dinner				
2 hr after				
Bedtime				

WEEK ....

DATE ....

Time	Monday	Tuesday	Wednesday	Thursday
Breakfast				
2 hr after				
Lunch				
2 hr after				
Dinner				
2 hr after				
Bedtime				

Time	Friday	Saturday	Sunday	NOTE
Breakfast				
2 hr after				
Lunch				
2 hr after				
Dinner				
2 hr after				
Bedtime				

WEEK ....

DATE ....

Time	Monday	Tuesday	Wednesday	Thursday
Breakfast				
2 hr after				
Lunch				
2 hr after				
Dinner				
2 hr after				
Bedtime				

Time	Friday	Saturday	Sunday	NOTE
Breakfast				
2 hr after				
Lunch				
2 hr after				
Dinner				
2 hr after				
Bedtime				

WEEK ....

DATE ....

Time	Monday	Tuesday	Wednesday	Thursday
Breakfast				
2 hr after				
Lunch				
2 hr after				
Dinner				
2 hr after				
Bedtime				

Time	Friday	Saturday	Sunday	NOTE
Breakfast				
2 hr after				
Lunch				
2 hr after				
Dinner				
2 hr after				
Bedtime				

WEEK ....

DATE ....

Time	Monday	Tuesday	Wednesday	Thursday
Breakfast				
2 hr after				
Lunch				
2 hr after				
Dinner				
2 hr after				
Bedtime				

Time	Friday	Saturday	Sunday	NOTE
Breakfast				
2 hr after				
Lunch				
2 hr after				
Dinner				
2 hr after				
Bedtime				

WEEK ....

DATE ....

Time	Monday	Tuesday	Wednesday	Thursday
Breakfast				
2 hr after				
Lunch				
2 hr after				
Dinner				
2 hr after				
Bedtime				

Time	Friday	Saturday	Sunday	NOTE
Breakfast				
2 hr after				
Lunch				
2 hr after				
Dinner				
2 hr after				
Bedtime				

WEEK ....

DATE ....

Time	Monday	Tuesday	Wednesday	Thursday
Breakfast				
2 hr after				
Lunch				
2 hr after				
Dinner				
2 hr after				
Bedtime				

Time	Friday	Saturday	Sunday	NOTE
Breakfast				
2 hr after				
Lunch				
2 hr after				
Dinner				
2 hr after				
Bedtime				

WEEK ....

DATE ....

Time	Monday	Tuesday	Wednesday	Thursday
Breakfast				
2 hr after				
Lunch				
2 hr after				
Dinner				
2 hr after				
Bedtime				

Time	Friday	Saturday	Sunday	NOTE
Breakfast				
2 hr after				
Lunch				
2 hr after				
Dinner				
2 hr after				
Bedtime				

WEEK ....

DATE ....

Time	Monday	Tuesday	Wednesday	Thursday
Breakfast				
2 hr after				
Lunch				
2 hr after				
Dinner				
2 hr after				
Bedtime				

Time	Friday	Saturday	Sunday	NOTE
Breakfast				
2 hr after				
Lunch				
2 hr after				
Dinner				
2 hr after				
Bedtime				

WEEK ....

DATE ....

Time	Monday	Tuesday	Wednesday	Thursday
Breakfast				
2 hr after				
Lunch				
2 hr after				
Dinner				
2 hr after				
Bedtime				

Time	Friday	Saturday	Sunday	NOTE
Breakfast				
2 hr after				
Lunch				
2 hr after				
Dinner				
2 hr after				
Bedtime				

WEEK ....

DATE ....

Time	Monday	Tuesday	Wednesday	Thursday
Breakfast				
2 hr after				
Lunch				
2 hr after				
Dinner				
2 hr after				
Bedtime				

Time	Friday	Saturday	Sunday	NOTE
Breakfast				
2 hr after				
Lunch				
2 hr after				
Dinner				
2 hr after				
Bedtime				

WEEK ....

DATE ....

Time	Monday	Tuesday	Wednesday	Thursday
Breakfast				
2 hr after				
Lunch				
2 hr after				
Dinner				
2 hr after				
Bedtime				

Time	Friday	Saturday	Sunday	NOTE
Breakfast				
2 hr after				
Lunch				
2 hr after				
Dinner				
2 hr after				
Bedtime				

WEEK ....

DATE ....

Time	Monday	Tuesday	Wednesday	Thursday
Breakfast				
2 hr after				
Lunch				
2 hr after				
Dinner				
2 hr after				
Bedtime				

Time	Friday	Saturday	Sunday	NOTE
Breakfast				
2 hr after				
Lunch				
2 hr after				
Dinner				
2 hr after				
Bedtime				

WEEK ....

DATE ....

Time	Monday	Tuesday	Wednesday	Thursday
Breakfast				
2 hr after				
Lunch				
2 hr after				
Dinner				
2 hr after				
Bedtime				

Time	Friday	Saturday	Sunday	NOTE
Breakfast				
2 hr after				
Lunch				
2 hr after				
Dinner				
2 hr after				
Bedtime				

WEEK ....

DATE ....

Time	Monday	Tuesday	Wednesday	Thursday
Breakfast				
2 hr after				
Lunch				
2 hr after				
Dinner				
2 hr after				
Bedtime				

Time	Friday	Saturday	Sunday	NOTE
Breakfast				
2 hr after				
Lunch				
2 hr after				
Dinner				
2 hr after				
Bedtime				

WEEK ....

DATE ....

Time	Monday	Tuesday	Wednesday	Thursday
Breakfast				
2 hr after				
Lunch				
2 hr after				
Dinner				
2 hr after				
Bedtime				

Time	Friday	Saturday	Sunday	NOTE
Breakfast				
2 hr after				
Lunch				
2 hr after				
Dinner				
2 hr after				
Bedtime				

WEEK ....

DATE ....

Time	Monday	Tuesday	Wednesday	Thursday
Breakfast				
2 hr after				
Lunch				
2 hr after				
Dinner				
2 hr after				
Bedtime				

Time	Friday	Saturday	Sunday	NOTE
Breakfast				
2 hr after				
Lunch				
2 hr after				
Dinner				
2 hr after				
Bedtime				

WEEK ....

DATE ....

Time	Monday	Tuesday	Wednesday	Thursday
Breakfast				
2 hr after				
Lunch				
2 hr after				
Dinner				
2 hr after				
Bedtime				

Time	Friday	Saturday	Sunday	NOTE
Breakfast				
2 hr after				
Lunch				
2 hr after				
Dinner				
2 hr after				
Bedtime				

WEEK ....

DATE ....

Time	Monday	Tuesday	Wednesday	Thursday
Breakfast				
2 hr after				
Lunch				
2 hr after				
Dinner				
2 hr after				
Bedtime				

Time	Friday	Saturday	Sunday	NOTE
Breakfast				
2 hr after				
Lunch				
2 hr after				
Dinner				
2 hr after				
Bedtime				

WEEK ....

DATE ....

Time	Monday	Tuesday	Wednesday	Thursday
Breakfast				
2 hr after				
Lunch				
2 hr after				
Dinner				
2 hr after				
Bedtime				

Time	Friday	Saturday	Sunday	NOTE
Breakfast				
2 hr after				
Lunch				
2 hr after				
Dinner				
2 hr after				
Bedtime				

WEEK ....

DATE ....

Time	Monday	Tuesday	Wednesday	Thursday
Breakfast				
2 hr after				
Lunch				
2 hr after				
Dinner				
2 hr after				
Bedtime				

Time	Friday	Saturday	Sunday	NOTE
Breakfast				
2 hr after				
Lunch				
2 hr after				
Dinner				
2 hr after				
Bedtime				

WEEK ....

DATE ....

Time	Monday	Tuesday	Wednesday	Thursday
Breakfast				
2 hr after				
Lunch				
2 hr after				
Dinner				
2 hr after				
Bedtime				

Time	Friday	Saturday	Sunday	NOTE
Breakfast				
2 hr after				
Lunch				
2 hr after				
Dinner				
2 hr after				
Bedtime				

WEEK ....

DATE ....

Time	Monday	Tuesday	Wednesday	Thursday
Breakfast				
2 hr after				
Lunch				
2 hr after				
Dinner				
2 hr after				
Bedtime				

Time	Friday	Saturday	Sunday	NOTE
Breakfast				
2 hr after				
Lunch				
2 hr after				
Dinner				
2 hr after				
Bedtime				

WEEK ....

DATE ....

Time	Monday	Tuesday	Wednesday	Thursday
Breakfast				
2 hr after				
Lunch				
2 hr after				
Dinner				
2 hr after				
Bedtime				

Time	Friday	Saturday	Sunday	NOTE
Breakfast				
2 hr after				
Lunch				
2 hr after				
Dinner				
2 hr after				
Bedtime				

WEEK ....

DATE ....

Time	Monday	Tuesday	Wednesday	Thursday
Breakfast				
2 hr after				
Lunch				
2 hr after				
Dinner				
2 hr after				
Bedtime				

Time	Friday	Saturday	Sunday	NOTE
Breakfast				
2 hr after				
Lunch				
2 hr after				
Dinner				
2 hr after				
Bedtime				

WEEK ....

DATE ....

Time	Monday	Tuesday	Wednesday	Thursday
Breakfast				
2 hr after				
Lunch				
2 hr after				
Dinner				
2 hr after				
Bedtime				

Time	Friday	Saturday	Sunday	NOTE
Breakfast				
2 hr after				
Lunch				
2 hr after				
Dinner				
2 hr after				
Bedtime				

WEEK ....

DATE ....

Time	Monday	Tuesday	Wednesday	Thursday
Breakfast				
2 hr after				
Lunch				
2 hr after				
Dinner				
2 hr after				
Bedtime				

Time	Friday	Saturday	Sunday	NOTE
Breakfast				
2 hr after				
Lunch				
2 hr after				
Dinner				
2 hr after				
Bedtime				

WEEK ....

DATE ....

Time	Monday	Tuesday	Wednesday	Thursday
Breakfast				
2 hr after				
Lunch				
2 hr after				
Dinner				
2 hr after				
Bedtime				

Time	Friday	Saturday	Sunday	NOTE
Breakfast				
2 hr after				
Lunch				
2 hr after				
Dinner				
2 hr after				
Bedtime				

WEEK ....

DATE ....

Time	Monday	Tuesday	Wednesday	Thursday
Breakfast				
2 hr after				
Lunch				
2 hr after				
Dinner				
2 hr after				
Bedtime				

Time	Friday	Saturday	Sunday	NOTE
Breakfast				
2 hr after				
Lunch				
2 hr after				
Dinner				
2 hr after				
Bedtime				

WEEK ....

DATE ....

Time	Monday	Tuesday	Wednesday	Thursday
Breakfast				
2 hr after				
Lunch				
2 hr after				
Dinner				
2 hr after				
Bedtime				

Time	Friday	Saturday	Sunday	NOTE
Breakfast				
2 hr after				
Lunch				
2 hr after				
Dinner				
2 hr after				
Bedtime				

WEEK ....

DATE ....

Time	Monday	Tuesday	Wednesday	Thursday
Breakfast				
2 hr after				
Lunch				
2 hr after				
Dinner				
2 hr after				
Bedtime				

Time	Friday	Saturday	Sunday	NOTE
Breakfast				
2 hr after				
Lunch				
2 hr after				
Dinner				
2 hr after				
Bedtime				

WEEK ....

DATE ....

Time	Monday	Tuesday	Wednesday	Thursday
Breakfast				
2 hr after				
Lunch				
2 hr after				
Dinner				
2 hr after				
Bedtime				

Time	Friday	Saturday	Sunday	NOTE
Breakfast				
2 hr after				
Lunch				
2 hr after				
Dinner				
2 hr after				
Bedtime				

WEEK ....

DATE ....

Time	Monday	Tuesday	Wednesday	Thursday
Breakfast				
2 hr after				
Lunch				
2 hr after				
Dinner				
2 hr after				
Bedtime				

Time	Friday	Saturday	Sunday	NOTE
Breakfast				
2 hr after				
Lunch				
2 hr after				
Dinner				
2 hr after				
Bedtime				

WEEK ....

DATE ....

Time	Monday	Tuesday	Wednesday	Thursday
Breakfast				
2 hr after				
Lunch				
2 hr after				
Dinner				
2 hr after				
Bedtime				

Time	Friday	Saturday	Sunday	NOTE
Breakfast				
2 hr after				
Lunch				
2 hr after				
Dinner				
2 hr after				
Bedtime				

WEEK ....

DATE ....

Time	Monday	Tuesday	Wednesday	Thursday
Breakfast				
2 hr after				
Lunch				
2 hr after				
Dinner				
2 hr after				
Bedtime				

Time	Friday	Saturday	Sunday	NOTE
Breakfast				
2 hr after				
Lunch				
2 hr after				
Dinner				
2 hr after				
Bedtime				

WEEK ....

DATE ....

Time	Monday	Tuesday	Wednesday	Thursday
Breakfast				
2 hr after				
Lunch				
2 hr after				
Dinner				
2 hr after				
Bedtime				

Time	Friday	Saturday	Sunday	NOTE
Breakfast				
2 hr after				
Lunch				
2 hr after				
Dinner				
2 hr after				
Bedtime				

WEEK ....

DATE ....

Time	Monday	Tuesday	Wednesday	Thursday
Breakfast				
2 hr after				
Lunch				
2 hr after				
Dinner				
2 hr after				
Bedtime				

Time	Friday	Saturday	Sunday	NOTE
Breakfast				
2 hr after				
Lunch				
2 hr after				
Dinner				
2 hr after				
Bedtime				

WEEK ....

DATE ....

Time	Monday	Tuesday	Wednesday	Thursday
Breakfast				
2 hr after				
Lunch				
2 hr after				
Dinner				
2 hr after				
Bedtime				

Time	Friday	Saturday	Sunday	NOTE
Breakfast				
2 hr after				
Lunch				
2 hr after				
Dinner				
2 hr after				
Bedtime				

WEEK ....

DATE ....

Time	Monday	Tuesday	Wednesday	Thursday
Breakfast				
2 hr after				
Lunch				
2 hr after				
Dinner				
2 hr after				
Bedtime				

Time	Friday	Saturday	Sunday	NOTE
Breakfast				
2 hr after				
Lunch				
2 hr after				
Dinner				
2 hr after				
Bedtime				

WEEK ....

DATE ....

Time	Monday	Tuesday	Wednesday	Thursday
Breakfast				
2 hr after				
Lunch				
2 hr after				
Dinner				
2 hr after				
Bedtime				

Time	Friday	Saturday	Sunday	NOTE
Breakfast				
2 hr after				
Lunch				
2 hr after				
Dinner				
2 hr after				
Bedtime				

WEEK ....

DATE ....

Time	Monday	Tuesday	Wednesday	Thursday
Breakfast				
2 hr after				
Lunch				
2 hr after				
Dinner				
2 hr after				
Bedtime				

Time	Friday	Saturday	Sunday	NOTE
Breakfast				
2 hr after				
Lunch				
2 hr after				
Dinner				
2 hr after				
Bedtime				

WEEK ....

DATE ....

Time	Monday	Tuesday	Wednesday	Thursday
Breakfast				
2 hr after				
Lunch				
2 hr after				
Dinner				
2 hr after				
Bedtime				

Time	Friday	Saturday	Sunday	NOTE
Breakfast				
2 hr after				
Lunch				
2 hr after				
Dinner				
2 hr after				
Bedtime				

WEEK ....

DATE ....

Time	Monday	Tuesday	Wednesday	Thursday
Breakfast				
2 hr after				
Lunch				
2 hr after				
Dinner				
2 hr after				
Bedtime				

Time	Friday	Saturday	Sunday	NOTE
Breakfast				
2 hr after				
Lunch				
2 hr after				
Dinner				
2 hr after				
Bedtime				

WEEK ....

DATE ....

Time	Monday	Tuesday	Wednesday	Thursday
Breakfast				
2 hr after				
Lunch				
2 hr after				
Dinner				
2 hr after				
Bedtime				

Time	Friday	Saturday	Sunday	NOTE
Breakfast				
2 hr after				
Lunch				
2 hr after				
Dinner				
2 hr after				
Bedtime				

WEEK ....

DATE ....

Time	Monday	Tuesday	Wednesday	Thursday
Breakfast				
2 hr after				
Lunch				
2 hr after				
Dinner				
2 hr after				
Bedtime				

Time	Friday	Saturday	Sunday	NOTE
Breakfast				
2 hr after				
Lunch				
2 hr after				
Dinner				
2 hr after				
Bedtime				

WEEK ....

DATE ....

Time	Monday	Tuesday	Wednesday	Thursday
Breakfast				
2 hr after				
Lunch				
2 hr after				
Dinner				
2 hr after				
Bedtime				

Time	Friday	Saturday	Sunday	NOTE
Breakfast				
2 hr after				
Lunch				
2 hr after				
Dinner				
2 hr after				
Bedtime				

WEEK ....

DATE ....

Time	Monday	Tuesday	Wednesday	Thursday
Breakfast				
2 hr after				
Lunch				
2 hr after				
Dinner				
2 hr after				
Bedtime				

Time	Friday	Saturday	Sunday	NOTE
Breakfast				
2 hr after				
Lunch				
2 hr after				
Dinner				
2 hr after				
Bedtime				

WEEK ....

DATE ....

Time	Monday	Tuesday	Wednesday	Thursday
Breakfast				
2 hr after				
Lunch				
2 hr after				
Dinner				
2 hr after				
Bedtime				

Time	Friday	Saturday	Sunday	NOTE
Breakfast				
2 hr after				
Lunch				
2 hr after				
Dinner				
2 hr after				
Bedtime				

WEEK ....

DATE ....

Time	Monday	Tuesday	Wednesday	Thursday
Breakfast				
2 hr after				
Lunch				
2 hr after				
Dinner				
2 hr after				
Bedtime				

Time	Friday	Saturday	Sunday	NOTE
Breakfast				
2 hr after				
Lunch				
2 hr after				
Dinner				
2 hr after				
Bedtime				

WEEK ....

DATE ....

Time	Monday	Tuesday	Wednesday	Thursday
Breakfast				
2 hr after				
Lunch				
2 hr after				
Dinner				
2 hr after				
Bedtime				

Time	Friday	Saturday	Sunday	NOTE
Breakfast				
2 hr after				
Lunch				
2 hr after				
Dinner				
2 hr after				
Bedtime				

WEEK ....

DATE ....

Time	Monday	Tuesday	Wednesday	Thursday
Breakfast				
2 hr after				
Lunch				
2 hr after				
Dinner				
2 hr after				
Bedtime				

Time	Friday	Saturday	Sunday	NOTE
Breakfast				
2 hr after				
Lunch				
2 hr after				
Dinner				
2 hr after				
Bedtime				

WEEK ....

DATE ....

Time	Monday	Tuesday	Wednesday	Thursday
Breakfast				
2 hr after				
Lunch				
2 hr after				
Dinner				
2 hr after				
Bedtime				

Time	Friday	Saturday	Sunday	NOTE
Breakfast				
2 hr after				
Lunch				
2 hr after				
Dinner				
2 hr after				
Bedtime				

WEEK ....

DATE ....

Time	Monday	Tuesday	Wednesday	Thursday
Breakfast				
2 hr after				
Lunch				
2 hr after				
Dinner				
2 hr after				
Bedtime				

Time	Friday	Saturday	Sunday	NOTE
Breakfast				
2 hr after				
Lunch				
2 hr after				
Dinner				
2 hr after				
Bedtime				

WEEK ....

DATE ....

Time	Monday	Tuesday	Wednesday	Thursday
Breakfast				
2 hr after				
Lunch				
2 hr after				
Dinner				
2 hr after				
Bedtime				

Time	Friday	Saturday	Sunday	NOTE
Breakfast				
2 hr after				
Lunch				
2 hr after				
Dinner				
2 hr after				
Bedtime				

WEEK ....

DATE ....

Time	Monday	Tuesday	Wednesday	Thursday
Breakfast				
2 hr after				
Lunch				
2 hr after				
Dinner				
2 hr after				
Bedtime				

Time	Friday	Saturday	Sunday	NOTE
Breakfast				
2 hr after				
Lunch				
2 hr after				
Dinner				
2 hr after				
Bedtime				

WEEK ....

DATE ....

Time	Monday	Tuesday	Wednesday	Thursday
Breakfast				
2 hr after				
Lunch				
2 hr after				
Dinner				
2 hr after				
Bedtime				

Time	Friday	Saturday	Sunday	NOTE
Breakfast				
2 hr after				
Lunch				
2 hr after				
Dinner				
2 hr after				
Bedtime				

WEEK ....

DATE ....

Time	Monday	Tuesday	Wednesday	Thursday
Breakfast				
2 hr after				
Lunch				
2 hr after				
Dinner				
2 hr after				
Bedtime				

Time	Friday	Saturday	Sunday	NOTE
Breakfast				
2 hr after				
Lunch				
2 hr after				
Dinner				
2 hr after				
Bedtime				

WEEK ....

DATE ....

Time	Monday	Tuesday	Wednesday	Thursday
Breakfast				
2 hr after				
Lunch				
2 hr after				
Dinner				
2 hr after				
Bedtime				

Time	Friday	Saturday	Sunday	NOTE
Breakfast				
2 hr after				
Lunch				
2 hr after				
Dinner				
2 hr after				
Bedtime				

WEEK ....

DATE ....

Time	Monday	Tuesday	Wednesday	Thursday
Breakfast				
2 hr after				
Lunch				
2 hr after				
Dinner				
2 hr after				
Bedtime				

Time	Friday	Saturday	Sunday	NOTE
Breakfast				
2 hr after				
Lunch				
2 hr after				
Dinner				
2 hr after				
Bedtime				

WEEK ....

DATE ....

Time	Monday	Tuesday	Wednesday	Thursday
Breakfast				
2 hr after				
Lunch				
2 hr after				
Dinner				
2 hr after				
Bedtime				

Time	Friday	Saturday	Sunday	NOTE
Breakfast				
2 hr after				
Lunch				
2 hr after				
Dinner				
2 hr after				
Bedtime				

WEEK ....

DATE ....

Time	Monday	Tuesday	Wednesday	Thursday
Breakfast				
2 hr after				
Lunch				
2 hr after				
Dinner				
2 hr after				
Bedtime				

Time	Friday	Saturday	Sunday	NOTE
Breakfast				
2 hr after				
Lunch				
2 hr after				
Dinner				
2 hr after				
Bedtime				

WEEK ....

DATE ....

Time	Monday	Tuesday	Wednesday	Thursday
Breakfast				
2 hr after				
Lunch				
2 hr after				
Dinner				
2 hr after				
Bedtime				

Time	Friday	Saturday	Sunday	NOTE
Breakfast				
2 hr after				
Lunch				
2 hr after				
Dinner				
2 hr after				
Bedtime				

WEEK ....

DATE ....

Time	Monday	Tuesday	Wednesday	Thursday
Breakfast				
2 hr after				
Lunch				
2 hr after				
Dinner				
2 hr after				
Bedtime				

Time	Friday	Saturday	Sunday	NOTE
Breakfast				
2 hr after				
Lunch				
2 hr after				
Dinner				
2 hr after				
Bedtime				

WEEK ....

DATE ....

Time	Monday	Tuesday	Wednesday	Thursday
Breakfast				
2 hr after				
Lunch				
2 hr after				
Dinner				
2 hr after				
Bedtime				

Time	Friday	Saturday	Sunday	NOTE
Breakfast				
2 hr after				
Lunch				
2 hr after				
Dinner				
2 hr after				
Bedtime				

WEEK ....

DATE ....

Time	Monday	Tuesday	Wednesday	Thursday
Breakfast				
2 hr after				
Lunch				
2 hr after				
Dinner				
2 hr after				
Bedtime				

Time	Friday	Saturday	Sunday	NOTE
Breakfast				
2 hr after				
Lunch				
2 hr after				
Dinner				
2 hr after				
Bedtime				

WEEK ....

DATE ....

Time	Monday	Tuesday	Wednesday	Thursday
Breakfast				
2 hr after				
Lunch				
2 hr after				
Dinner				
2 hr after				
Bedtime				

Time	Friday	Saturday	Sunday	NOTE
Breakfast				
2 hr after				
Lunch				
2 hr after				
Dinner				
2 hr after				
Bedtime				

WEEK ....

DATE ....

Time	Monday	Tuesday	Wednesday	Thursday
Breakfast				
2 hr after				
Lunch				
2 hr after				
Dinner				
2 hr after				
Bedtime				

Time	Friday	Saturday	Sunday	NOTE
Breakfast				
2 hr after				
Lunch				
2 hr after				
Dinner				
2 hr after				
Bedtime				

WEEK ....

DATE ....

Time	Monday	Tuesday	Wednesday	Thursday
Breakfast				
2 hr after				
Lunch				
2 hr after				
Dinner				
2 hr after				
Bedtime				

Time	Friday	Saturday	Sunday	NOTE
Breakfast				
2 hr after				
Lunch				
2 hr after				
Dinner				
2 hr after				
Bedtime				

WEEK ....

DATE ....

Time	Monday	Tuesday	Wednesday	Thursday
Breakfast				
2 hr after				
Lunch				
2 hr after				
Dinner				
2 hr after				
Bedtime				

Time	Friday	Saturday	Sunday	NOTE
Breakfast				
2 hr after				
Lunch				
2 hr after				
Dinner				
2 hr after				
Bedtime				

WEEK ....

DATE ....

Time	Monday	Tuesday	Wednesday	Thursday
Breakfast				
2 hr after				
Lunch				
2 hr after				
Dinner				
2 hr after				
Bedtime				

Time	Friday	Saturday	Sunday	NOTE
Breakfast				
2 hr after				
Lunch				
2 hr after				
Dinner				
2 hr after				
Bedtime				

WEEK ....

DATE ....

Time	Monday	Tuesday	Wednesday	Thursday
Breakfast				
2 hr after				
Lunch				
2 hr after				
Dinner				
2 hr after				
Bedtime				

Time	Friday	Saturday	Sunday	NOTE
Breakfast				
2 hr after				
Lunch				
2 hr after				
Dinner				
2 hr after				
Bedtime				

WEEK ....

DATE ....

Time	Monday	Tuesday	Wednesday	Thursday
Breakfast				
2 hr after				
Lunch				
2 hr after				
Dinner				
2 hr after				
Bedtime				

Time	Friday	Saturday	Sunday	NOTE
Breakfast				
2 hr after				
Lunch				
2 hr after				
Dinner				
2 hr after				
Bedtime				

WEEK ....

DATE ....

Time	Monday	Tuesday	Wednesday	Thursday
Breakfast				
2 hr after				
Lunch				
2 hr after				
Dinner				
2 hr after				
Bedtime				

Time	Friday	Saturday	Sunday	NOTE
Breakfast				
2 hr after				
Lunch				
2 hr after				
Dinner				
2 hr after				
Bedtime				

WEEK ....

DATE ....

Time	Monday	Tuesday	Wednesday	Thursday
Breakfast				
2 hr after				
Lunch				
2 hr after				
Dinner				
2 hr after				
Bedtime				

Time	Friday	Saturday	Sunday	NOTE
Breakfast				
2 hr after				
Lunch				
2 hr after				
Dinner				
2 hr after				
Bedtime				

WEEK ....

DATE ....

Time	Monday	Tuesday	Wednesday	Thursday
Breakfast				
2 hr after				
Lunch				
2 hr after				
Dinner				
2 hr after				
Bedtime				

Time	Friday	Saturday	Sunday	NOTE
Breakfast				
2 hr after				
Lunch				
2 hr after				
Dinner				
2 hr after				
Bedtime				

WEEK ....

DATE ....

Time	Monday	Tuesday	Wednesday	Thursday
Breakfast				
2 hr after				
Lunch				
2 hr after				
Dinner				
2 hr after				
Bedtime				

Time	Friday	Saturday	Sunday	NOTE
Breakfast				
2 hr after				
Lunch				
2 hr after				
Dinner				
2 hr after				
Bedtime				

WEEK ....

DATE ....

Time	Monday	Tuesday	Wednesday	Thursday
Breakfast				
2 hr after				
Lunch				
2 hr after				
Dinner				
2 hr after				
Bedtime				

Time	Friday	Saturday	Sunday	NOTE
Breakfast				
2 hr after				
Lunch				
2 hr after				
Dinner				
2 hr after				
Bedtime				

WEEK ....

DATE ....

Time	Monday	Tuesday	Wednesday	Thursday
Breakfast				
2 hr after				
Lunch				
2 hr after				
Dinner				
2 hr after				
Bedtime				

Time	Friday	Saturday	Sunday	NOTE
Breakfast				
2 hr after				
Lunch				
2 hr after				
Dinner				
2 hr after				
Bedtime				

WEEK ....

DATE ....

Time	Monday	Tuesday	Wednesday	Thursday
Breakfast				
2 hr after				
Lunch				
2 hr after				
Dinner				
2 hr after				
Bedtime				

Time	Friday	Saturday	Sunday	NOTE
Breakfast				
2 hr after				
Lunch				
2 hr after				
Dinner				
2 hr after				
Bedtime				

WEEK ....

DATE ....

Time	Monday	Tuesday	Wednesday	Thursday
Breakfast				
2 hr after				
Lunch				
2 hr after				
Dinner				
2 hr after				
Bedtime				

Time	Friday	Saturday	Sunday	NOTE
Breakfast				
2 hr after				
Lunch				
2 hr after				
Dinner				
2 hr after				
Bedtime				

WEEK ....

DATE ....

Time	Monday	Tuesday	Wednesday	Thursday
Breakfast				
2 hr after				
Lunch				
2 hr after				
Dinner				
2 hr after				
Bedtime				

Time	Friday	Saturday	Sunday	NOTE
Breakfast				
2 hr after				
Lunch				
2 hr after				
Dinner				
2 hr after				
Bedtime				

WEEK ....

DATE ....

Time	Monday	Tuesday	Wednesday	Thursday
Breakfast				
2 hr after				
Lunch				
2 hr after				
Dinner				
2 hr after				
Bedtime				

Time	Friday	Saturday	Sunday	NOTE
Breakfast				
2 hr after				
Lunch				
2 hr after				
Dinner				
2 hr after				
Bedtime				

WEEK ....

DATE ....

Time	Monday	Tuesday	Wednesday	Thursday
Breakfast				
2 hr after				
Lunch				
2 hr after				
Dinner				
2 hr after				
Bedtime				

Time	Friday	Saturday	Sunday	NOTE
Breakfast				
2 hr after				
Lunch				
2 hr after				
Dinner				
2 hr after				
Bedtime				

WEEK ....

DATE ....

Time	Monday	Tuesday	Wednesday	Thursday
Breakfast				
2 hr after				
Lunch				
2 hr after				
Dinner				
2 hr after				
Bedtime				

Time	Friday	Saturday	Sunday	NOTE
Breakfast				
2 hr after				
Lunch				
2 hr after				
Dinner				
2 hr after				
Bedtime				

WEEK ....

DATE ....

Time	Monday	Tuesday	Wednesday	Thursday
Breakfast				
2 hr after				
Lunch				
2 hr after				
Dinner				
2 hr after				
Bedtime				

Time	Friday	Saturday	Sunday	NOTE
Breakfast				
2 hr after				
Lunch				
2 hr after				
Dinner				
2 hr after				
Bedtime				

WEEK ....

DATE ....

Time	Monday	Tuesday	Wednesday	Thursday
Breakfast				
2 hr after				
Lunch				
2 hr after				
Dinner				
2 hr after				
Bedtime				

Time	Friday	Saturday	Sunday	NOTE
Breakfast				
2 hr after				
Lunch				
2 hr after				
Dinner				
2 hr after				
Bedtime				

WEEK ....

DATE ....

Time	Monday	Tuesday	Wednesday	Thursday
Breakfast				
2 hr after				
Lunch				
2 hr after				
Dinner				
2 hr after				
Bedtime				

Time	Friday	Saturday	Sunday	NOTE
Breakfast				
2 hr after				
Lunch				
2 hr after				
Dinner				
2 hr after				
Bedtime				

WEEK ....

DATE ....

Time	Monday	Tuesday	Wednesday	Thursday
Breakfast				
2 hr after				
Lunch				
2 hr after				
Dinner				
2 hr after				
Bedtime				

Time	Friday	Saturday	Sunday	NOTE
Breakfast				
2 hr after				
Lunch				
2 hr after				
Dinner				
2 hr after				
Bedtime				

WEEK ....

DATE ....

Time	Monday	Tuesday	Wednesday	Thursday
Breakfast				
2 hr after				
Lunch				
2 hr after				
Dinner				
2 hr after				
Bedtime				

Time	Friday	Saturday	Sunday	NOTE
Breakfast				
2 hr after				
Lunch				
2 hr after				
Dinner				
2 hr after				
Bedtime				

WEEK ....

DATE ....

Time	Monday	Tuesday	Wednesday	Thursday
Breakfast				
2 hr after				
Lunch				
2 hr after				
Dinner				
2 hr after				
Bedtime				

Time	Friday	Saturday	Sunday	NOTE
Breakfast				
2 hr after				
Lunch				
2 hr after				
Dinner				
2 hr after				
Bedtime